I wish masks worked.

I wish masks worked. If they did they'd be a cheap, easy way to slow the spread of Sars-Cov-2.

I wish masks worked. The idea they protect not just their wearers but also the people around them seems wonderfully selfless.

I wish masks worked. Americans are spending billions of dollars on them and they can cause acne and frighten small children and people with disabilities. Wearing them for no reason seems perverse.

I wish masks worked. Most Americans now wear them. Telling people they have been conned doesn't make them happy.

I wish masks worked. They have become *the* flashpoint in the political battles around Sars-Cov-2. Anyone who opposes wearing masks, much less making everyone wear them, draws scorn from the media and scientific establishment. *Bet you think the virus is fake, too. People are dying!*

I wish masks worked. We have so many other battles to fight around coronavirus: lockdowns, school closings, travel restrictions, and other government intrusions into our lives. Masks seem at first like one that isn't worth the trouble. *Wear a mask,* the advocates insist. *Stop arguing, just wear it. It's nothing.*

I wish masks worked.

D0150299

But they don't.

Not the ordinary cloth and surgical masks that nearly everybody wears, anyway. Despite everything the media and public health experts have told you, *they don't work.*

More accurately, we have no real evidence they do – and plenty of evidence they don't.

Welcome to Part 3 of Unreported Truths: masks. As protection, masks are largely useless, and mask mandates even more so. But as a symbol that the coronavirus is a serious danger requiring us to give up our rights, they are incredibly effective.

A lot has happened since the last installment came out in August. President Trump was infected with Sars-Cov-2 and recovered. A new outbreak raced across Europe and the United States. Several drug and biotechnology companies announced positive results for vaccines.

And Joe Biden narrowly won the presidential election, eking out a coin flip win over Donald Trump. (Whatever you think of mail-in ballots, Republicans have found no evidence of large-scale vote fraud. We should all assume Biden will take the oath of office in January.)

Elections have consequences, Barack Obama famously said. The 2020 presidential election surely will, especially for the way we respond to the coronavirus.

Biden, who was rarely photographed without a mask during the campaign, has already promised to try to make all Americans wear masks. "We can save tens of thousands of lives if everyone would just wear a mask," he said at a press conference on Nov. 9.

(https://www.nbcnews.com/politics/2020-election/biden-kicks-presidential-transition-begging-americans-wear-masks-n1247143)

Biden's official Website, "Buildbackbetter.com," calls for:

"Every American to wear a mask when they are around people outside their household.

"Every Governor to make that mandatory in their state.

"Local authorities to also make it mandatory to buttress their state orders."

Biden's proposal makes no distinction between requiring masks indoors and outdoors, or only when strangers are close together. Its language suggests Biden wants to force all of us to wear masks all the time, except when we are home with only family members around.

Biden's win also emboldened public health authorities to press masks even harder. A week after Election Day, the Centers for Disease Control issued a new advisory in which it claimed even cloth masks reduce the risk of infection in the people who wear them. The CDC wrote:

> Masks are primarily intended to reduce the emission of virus-laden droplets ("source control")... Masks also help reduce inhalation of these droplets by the wearer ("filtration for personal protection").

(https://www.cdc.gov/coronavirus/2019-ncov/more/masking-science-sars-cov2.html)

The CDC's promise that cloth and surgical masks protect the people wearing them is notable. It stands in marked contrast to what pro-mask epidemiologists have said since April. Usually, they focus on the protection masks supposedly offer to *other* people ("My mask protects you, your mask protects me.")

So why the change? The CDC decided to talk up personal protection in the hope of convincing people who aren't wearing masks to do so, according to NBC News:

> Infectious disease doctors who have urged the CDC to change the messaging around masks believe it will be a more effective public health strategy. "I'm thrilled that it's happening now," said Dr. Monica Gandhi, professor of medicine at the University of California San Francisco. "I think it helps people comply with the regulation if they think it's helping them."

(https://www.nbcnews.com/health/health-news/two-way-street-cdc-report-says-masks-protect-wearers-everyone-n1247258)

The not very well-hidden subtext here: People who are too selfish to wear masks to protect *others* might do so for their own safety.

Biden's request for *local* governments to press for mandatory mask-wearing is also notable. For the most part, states have led the push for masks, focusing on businesses rather than individuals. State health departments now make stores, restaurants, and offices require masks for entry. But local police departments have generally avoided arresting people for going maskless. The mention of "local authorities" looks to be Biden's backdoor way to change that.

Still, law enforcement is not the main driver of mask use. Public pressure is.

Ironically, in February and March, as the epidemic was taking off, the pressure came the other way. Health experts discouraged the public from using face coverings. On Feb. 29,

Dr. Jerome Adams, the Surgeon General, tweeted a warning that would become infamous:

> Seriously people — STOP BUYING MASKS! They are NOT effective in preventing general public from catching #Coronavirus, but if healthcare providers can't get them to care for sick patients, it puts them and our communities at risk!

A week later, on March 8, Dr. Anthony Fauci, the director of the National Institute of Allergy and Infectious Diseases, told 60 Minutes:

> There's no reason to be walking around with a mask. When you're in the middle of an outbreak, wearing a mask might make people feel a little bit better and it might even block a droplet, but it's not providing the perfect protection that people think that it is. And, often, there are unintended consequences — people keep fiddling with the mask and they keep touching their face."

The World Health Organization also warned against wearing masks. "WHO stands by recommendation to not wear masks if you are not sick or not caring for someone who is sick," CNN reported on March 30.

---

[1](https://twitter.com/surgeon_general/status/1233725785283932160?lang=en)

(https://www.reuters.com/article/uk-factcheck-fauci-outdated-video-masks/fact-checkoutdated-video-of-fauci-saying-theres-no-reason-to-be-walking-around-with-a-mask-idUSKBN26T2TR)

(https://www.cnn.com/2020/03/30/world/coronavirus-who-masks-recommendation-trnd/index.html)

(https://www.nejm.org/doi/full/10.1056/NEJMp2006372)

On April 1, the *New England Journal of Medicine* – the leading American health-care journal – wrote:

> We know that wearing a mask outside health care facilities offers little, if any, protection from infection... In many cases, the desire for widespread masking is a reflexive reaction to anxiety over the pandemic.[1]

But within days of that article, health experts reversed course and insisted people must wear masks – whether they were feeling sick or well, whether they were in hospitals or stores or even outside.

On April 22, Dr. Adams – he of "STOP BUYING MASKS" – unveiled the new mantra at a White House press conference: "You wear your mask to protect me... I wear my mask to protect you."

(https://www.whitehouse.gov/briefings-statements/remarks-president-trump-vice-president-pence-members-coronavirus-task-force-press-briefing-30/)

As states rolled back lockdowns in May and June, the advice became more strident. Masks were now the most important step to slow the epidemic. Face coverings were crucial not just for people with Covid but for those without, because even people without symptoms could spread the disease.

By June 3, the authors of the April 1 New England Journal of Medicine were claiming readers had misunderstood their original piece:

> We understand that some people are citing our Perspective article... as support for discrediting widespread masking. In truth, the intent of our article was to push for more masking, not less.

(https://www.nejm.org/doi/full/10.1056/NEJMc2020836)

Sure. The statement that masks outside hospitals offer *"little if any protection from infection"* was meant to encourage their use.

But the same media outlets which failed to ask questions about the need for lockdowns were just as credulous on the sudden 180-degree turn over masks. News organizations happily accepted the excuse by public health authorities that they had initially offered anti-mask advice only to prevent a run on masks that healthcare workers needed. In newspapers and on cable networks, pro-mask messages became the norm.

"Overnight, masks have become a symbol of social responsibility," The New York Times wrote on April 10. "If you still need convincing, here's why you now should be wearing a mask in public spaces." Two months later, the Times cheerily offered "Tips for Making Your Mask Work."

The Washington Post took slightly longer. On April 17, it called mask-wearing a "tough decision" and noted many states had originally enacted anti-mask laws to combat the Ku Klux Klan. On May 1, it warned that masks could cause painful rashes and acne for their wearers:

---

[2] https://www.nytimes.com/2020/04/10/well/live/coronavirus-face-masks-guides-protection-personal-protective-equipment.html

https://www.nytimes.com/interactive/2020/06/25/burst/how-to-get-the-most-out-of-your-mask.html

https://www.washingtonpost.com/health/tips-on-alleviating-face-masks-rashes-and-skin-irritations/2020/05/01/5dd3f2ac-88b0-11ea-ac8a-fe9b8088e101_story.html

https://www.washingtonpost.com/health/2020/06/13/spate-new-research-supports-wearing-masks-control-coronavirus-spread/

> Skin irritation from wearing personal protective equipment is a hazard already familiar to health-care providers working in settings where infection control is critical. Now it has also become familiar to many people wearing masks in public.

But by June, the Post was fully on board, explaining how "new research supports wearing masks to control coronavirus spread."[2]

The next step followed logically.

Having decreed masks could save people from Sars-Cov-2, media outlets tried to embarrass anyone who refused. Not to wear a mask was to refuse to "follow the science" – a catchphrase repeated endlessly – and a sign of selfishness.

Newspapers and magazines published insufferably arrogant pieces telling readers how to deal with the cretins who wouldn't wear masks. "It can be difficult to find common ground with someone who refuses to wear a mask for whatever reason," Teen Vogue wrote in July. "You might find the most resistance from people who are ideologically opposed to wearing masks because they believe doing so is a sign of weakness (it isn't)."

(https://www.teenvogue.com/story/how-to-talk-to-people-who-wont-wear-face-masks)

The Washington Post went a step further, warning in September, "Some Covid-19 rule-breakers could be narcissists, experts say. Here's how to approach them – " as if people who'd decided to keep their faces uncovered were inherently dangerous. The article even offered strategies to approach those awful narcissists. Craig Malkin, a psychologist, suggested telling them how important they were:

> "For example, [say] 'You can make the difference between life and death because we're all in this together.'"

> "The less significant they feel in all of this, the more they're going to have to pound their chests and push back against what's being expected to feel like they matter," Malkin said.

(https://www.washingtonpost.com/lifestyle/wellness/narcissism-mask-covid-psychology/2020/09/25/d3de1b32-fe9c-11ea-9ceb-061d646d9c67_story.html)

In August, a study would take this argument to the extreme. People who didn't wear masks were no longer just dumb or self-centered. They were sociopaths:

> New research from Brazil has found that people who are unconcerned with adhering to measures to prevent the spread of Covid-19 tend to display higher levels of traits associated with antisocial personality disorder, also known as sociopathy.

(https://www.news-medical.net/news/20200824/Sociopaths-less-likely-to-comply-with-COVID-mask-hygiene-and-social-distancing.aspx)

The relentless pressure has caused a sharp rise in mask wearing. In blue states like California, masks are essentially standard, even outside. People who wear masks are increasingly willing to challenge people who don't. I live in New York and try not to wear a mask outside, so I have seen the change in attitudes firsthand. Recently, a masked woman in her sixties asked me if I would step aside since she needed to walk around me and I wasn't wearing a mask. We were standing several feet apart on a hiking trail.

National surveys confirm mask wearing has risen substantially. In June, about 65 percent of Americans said they wore masks in stores all or most of the time, according to Pew Research. By August the figure had risen to 85 percent.

(https://www.pewresearch.org/fact-tank/2020/08/27/more-americans-say-they-are-regularly-wearing-masks-in-stores-and-other-businesses/)

Other surveys show even more mask use.

Those percentages might slightly overstate real-world mask wearing, for the same reason polls understated Trump's support. People don't like to admit they deviate from media-promoted social norms. Still, mask wearing is clearly now the default, indoors everywhere and outdoors in most states.

Which is why it may be so surprising that the United States is now going through its third and apparently largest wave of coronavirus infections. The first and second epidemics were largely regional: the spring wave in the Northeast and Midwest, the summer outbreak in the Sunbelt. The fall outbreak seems to be everywhere. The number of reported infections – which the media calls "cases," though they are based mainly on test results and include many people with no symptoms – has reached record highs.

The number of positive tests overstates the scope of the fall epidemic because the United States now tests more than 10 million people a week, far more than it did during the spring. Further, many positive tests represent people who *had* rather than currently have Sars-Cov-2 infections. (I may address the details of the issues around PCR tests in a future booklet; they are technical but crucially important.)

Still, hospitalizations are also rising. More than 80,000 Americans are now hospitalized with the coronavirus, more than the spring or summer peaks. The growth in testing is partially driving that rise. A significant fraction of those patients have been hospitalized for other problems. They are then found to be infected with Sars-Cov-2 when they are tested in the hospital.

But part of the increase in hospitalizations is real. And some regional hospital networks are under strain. The evidence is clear: the coronavirus is spreading faster in the United States than it has in months.

All by itself this fact should raise serious questions about how well masks prevent the transmission of the coronavirus. Health authorities have told Americans for six months to wear masks. We have listened. More of us are wearing masks more often than ever before. Yet the virus is spreading faster.

How can that be, if masks work?

2

The answer is that the evidence that face coverings do any good turns out to be even more porous than masks themselves.

Understanding why requires some background in the biology of viruses and the ways they spread.

Figuring out how Sars-Cov-2 – or any respiratory virus – jumps between people is very complicated. Figuring out if masks reduce transmission is even more so. Some of the language scientists use adds to the confusion in ways that make masks seem more effective than they are.

We know Sars-Cov-2 spreads mainly through the air. Transmission through touching "fomites" on contaminated surfaces is less common than was initially thought. Infected people exhale viral particles – virions – that are usually carried inside larger molecules made mostly of water and called "aerosols" or "droplets." People around the infected person inhale those aerosols or droplets and are exposed to the virus.

The distinction between an aerosol and a droplet is size: aerosols are smaller. But the word "droplet" doesn't mean what it seems to mean. It does *not* imply a raindrop-sized visible particle, like a mucus ball that a person with a cold might blow into a handkerchief.

An average raindrop is about 1/25th of an inch, or 1 millimeter – 1/1000th of a meter. Most people can't see objects smaller than about 0.1 millimeters without using a magnifying glass or microscope.

Viruses, aerosols, and droplets are measured on much smaller scales.

Below a millimeter, the next common unit of length is the micrometer or micron. A micron is 1/1000th of a millimeter, or 1/1,000,000th of a meter. The smallest object people can see – 0.1 millimeters – equals 100 microns.

When scientists talk about "droplets," they mean any exhaled particle more than 5 microns, 1/5000th of an inch, far too small for anyone to see unaided. Aerosols are even smaller – less than 5 microns.

The coronavirus itself is smaller still. For it, scientists use still another measure of length, the nanometer. 1 nanometer is 1/1000th of a micron. In other words, 1 meter equals one *billion* nanometers. An average-sized man is about 1,700,000,000 nanometers tall.

But a single virion of Sars-Cov-2 is about 60 to 140 nanometers, or 0.1 microns.

The different measurement scales can be confusing.

But the first takeaway is simple. Whatever masks do – or don't do – to protect us from the coronavirus is mostly *invisible.* Masks can obviously catch visible chunks of spit or phlegm, but the virus mostly travels on much smaller particles.

The second takeaway is also simple. All masks are not created equal, even if they all look more or less the same. For a mask to provide decent protection, it must be made of a material fine enough to catch nearly all of those tiny aerosols and droplets.

Such face coverings do exist.

Technically, they aren't called masks at all, but respirators.

Respirators must be certified as offering specific levels of protection before they're sold. In the United States, the most common models are called N95s. They have that name because manufacturers must prove they catch at least 95 percent of all particles of 300 nanometers – 0.3 microns. Many N95 masks prove even more effective than that standard in laboratory testing, blocking up to 99 percent of all but the smallest particles.

In contrast, standards for surgical masks are far less strict, and standards for homemade cloth masks don't exist. (Surgical masks are often light blue and made of three layers. The inside and outside are non-woven fabric, the middle a thin melted plastic layer, usually polypropylene. Cloth masks can be made of almost any fabric and can be one or multiple layers. Most Americans now seem to wear cloth masks in public, though surgical masks are also common.)

Further, unlike ordinary masks, N95 respirators are supposed to be "fit-tested." In other words, they're meant to attach tightly to the face of the person wearing them, with no gaps that allow unfiltered air between their edges and the skin. "The respirator must fit the user's face snugly (i.e., create a seal," the Centers for Disease Control wrote in an advisory about masks in March.

(https://blogs.cdc.gov/niosh-science-blog/2020/03/16/n95-preparedness/)

But ordinary masks are not fit-tested. Sometimes they are tied over the ear. More frequently they come with preattached loops. So ordinary masks start with two huge disadvantages compared to N95s. Their material offers less protection, *and* they don't fit as well.

But N95s are expensive, and even trained medical staff dislike wearing them for more than a few hours. As two doctors wrote in a commentary in August, "when worn properly, N95 masks are suffocating, uncomfortable, and difficult to tolerate for long durations."

(https://jamanetwork.com/journals/jamainternalmedicine/fullarticle/2769441)

As a practical matter, if civilians are going to wear face coverings, they will be standard cloth or surgical masks. But the limitations of those masks were well documented long before the coronavirus epidemic.

In 2009, four researchers examined how well surgical masks worked to filter small particles, those of 1 micron (1000 nanometers) or less. Their conclusion: badly.

In a paper called "Filtration Performance of FDA-Cleared Surgical Masks," the scientists tested five surgical mask brands. Four of the five masks allowed 15 percent or more of 100-nanometer (virus-sized) to 1 micron-sized particles through. Two of the five allowed more than half of those particles through.

Making matters worse, the authors believed their results actually overstated the real-world performance of the masks. They had sealed their masks to the "faces" of their mannikins with silicone. "A surgical mask user would be expected to get protection levels far less than that observed in this study, because a complete sealing of a surgical mask to a human face cannot be achieved," they wrote.

They concluded with a warning: "The wide variation in penetration levels for room air particles, which included particles in the same size range of viruses, confirms that **surgical masks should not be used for respiratory protection** [emphasis added]."

(https://www.ncbi.nlm.nih.gov/pmc/articles/PMC7357397/)

More recent studies have also found surgical masks were mostly ineffective compared to N95s.

One paper was published in August and focused on the question of whether expired N95s were still safe to use. On that issue, the researchers found good news. Long after their posted expiration dates, most N95s still worked.

But as part of the study, the researchers also checked the performance of surgical masks. And they used human subjects rather than mannikins, for a more realistic demonstration of the way masks fit.

The scientists found the surgical masks barely worked. Masks with ties filtered about 70 percent of small particles. Those with ear loops filtered less than 40 percent and often had "visible gaps between the face mask and the wearer."

(Dr. Michael Osterholm, an infectious disease expert, made the same point more graphically in a June podcast interview. Based on the pictures he saw of people wearing masks, about one person in four was wearing them wrongly, the equivalent "of fixing three of the five screen doors on your submarine." Rather than masks, Osterholm said he preferred to focus on encouraging people to stay at least six feet apart.[3])

The August paper makes clear that – if a shortage of new N95s forces them to choose – health-care workers should pick old N95s over new surgical masks. But the authors didn't explicitly say so in their conclusion, maybe because they were aware that *any* criticism of masks is off-limits in the coronavirus era.

Instead, they pointed out that their work offered "quantitative results... [for] evidence-based decisions."

[3] https://www.ama-assn.org/delivering-care/public-health/covid-19-s-first-wave-may-be-only-wave-no-pause)

In other words, *we're not going to tell you surgical masks don't work – you can read.*

What's true for surgical masks appears to be doubly true for homemade cloth masks, which generally filter even fewer small particles and are even *less* effective. The overall evidence is clear: Standard cloth and surgical masks offer next to no protection against virus-sized particles or small aerosols.

But maybe that failure doesn't matter. Can we be sure that the virus actually floats in particles that small?

Yes.

In a paper published in the November International Journal of Infectious Diseases, a team of researchers reported finding Sars-Cov-2 viral particles floating in the air of a hospital room. The virus they collected could reproduce in cell cultures – meaning it was "alive," not merely dead fragments of viral particles.

In their conclusion, the researchers explained:

> The public health implications are broad, particularly as current best practices for limiting the spread of COVID-19 center on social distancing, **wearing of face coverings while in proximity to others** [emphasis added] and hand washing. For aerosol-based transmission, measures such as physical distancing by 6 feet would not be helpful in an indoor setting, provide a false sense of security, and lead to exposures and outbreaks.

Once again, the researchers didn't explicitly say that if physical distancing "would not be helpful" against aerosol-based transmission, *masks* also wouldn't be. Such is the pressure to encourage mask wearing.

(https://www.sciencedirect.com/science/article/pii/S1201971220307396)

The fact dormitories, prisons, ships, and other "congregate" settings can see very high rates of coronavirus infection – as high as 90 percent – also provides strong real-world evidence that Sars-Cov-2 spreads through tiny aerosol particles that stay in the air for long periods. Person-to-person transmission would be unlikely to spread the virus that quickly or effectively.

In one study of coronavirus transmission in a San Francisco homeless shelter, researchers found that they could track only four "close contacts" to the two original cases at the shelter, and 18 people in beds within six feet. But in testing only three to four days after the initial positive tests from the first two cases, 101 residents of the shelter tested positive. At the time, San Francisco had very low community transmission of Sars-Cov-2, so it is likely the residents were infected inside the shelter.

(https://www.ncbi.nlm.nih.gov/pmc/articles/PMC7454344/)

In fact, as early as February, Chinese health authorities warned that "aerosol transmission" was a major transmission route. They urged people to keep windows open.
(https://www.chinadaily.com.cn/a/202002/08/WS5e3e7d97a310128217275fc3.html)

The theoretical evidence that cloth and surgical masks do not protect their wearers is overwhelming. But we have even *stronger* evidence. It comes from real-world clinical trials of people wearing masks.

Medical proof comes in many different forms.

The weakest evidence comes from anecdotes based on one person's experience. Just because I didn't have an accident after driving drunk doesn't mean doing so is safe.

On the other hand, the gold standard of evidence comes from what scientists and physicians call randomized controlled trials. In those trials, researchers recruit people and split them into evenly matched groups. They then offer one group a certain treatment and another no treatment.

Suppose I believe a cholesterol-lowering drug called a statin can reduce heart disease. I give some of the people in my trial the statin and the rest a placebo pill that contains no medicine. When the trial is over, I check whether the people who took the statin had fewer heart attacks and strokes than the ones who received the placebo pill. If they did, I can assume the statin is responsible for the difference. In fact, companies and independent researchers have run many such trials and consistently found statins reduce heart disease. So if you have high cholesterol, your doctor will prescribe a statin.

But it's crucial to remember that even if I have reason to think a treatment will work, *unless I run the trial I don't know.* Drug companies spent billions of dollars on another kind of cholesterol-lowering medicine called a CETP inhibitor. But when they tested those drugs in clinical trials, they found deaths *rose.* They had to quit developing them.

Even a good idea can fail in practice, which is why the four most important words in medicine are *"First, do no harm."* For centuries, well-meaning physicians used techniques we find horrifying today, in part because they depended on anecdotal evidence and hope rather than hard data from clinical trials.

Anecdotes are on one end; clinical trial evidence is on the other. A huge variety of data exists between the two. Some is what scientists call pre-clinical, like "in vitro" studies on cells in laboratories, or animal research, or mechanistic studies designed to show how and why a treatment might work. All those studies should be viewed with caution. No one can be sure how lab results will translate into humans. Cancer researchers often joke that they've cured tumors many times – in mice.

Another form of evidence is real-world data in people that doesn't come out of a clinical trial.

For example, researchers might track whether people who have quit drinking are less likely to start again if they go to Alcoholics Anonymous meetings. Or they might try to figure out what's causing changes in even larger groups. Why have car accidents risen in one state but not another? We call this kind of work epidemiology – trying to measure and control diseases and dangerous behaviors in groups of people.

But this research has a huge caveat. Unless they set up the groups in advance, researchers cannot know if the people in the two groups were truly the same going in. So they can't be sure what has caused the changes they see.

In the AA example, maybe the people who went to AA meetings seem less likely to drink again *because they were so motivated to stop drinking that they went to meetings,* not because of any help the meetings themselves provide. Or maybe not – maybe the meetings actually work. (Addiction researchers have debated this issue for decades.)

Worse, as the groups get bigger and more diverse, researchers will have a harder and harder time figuring out what's really causing the changes.

Thus when we're trying to figure out whether a treatment actually works, the best evidence by far comes from clinical trials. Nothing else comes close.

And clinical trials consistently find that masks *don't* protect people from respiratory viruses.

In February, seven researchers in Hong Kong reviewed *all* the trials they could find that tested whether masks outside hospital settings protected their wearers against the flu. They found 10 studies that had been conducted since 1946. (The number is relatively small, given the importance of the question. The reason is that trials are expensive. Prescription drug companies, which pay for most of them, have no incentive to spend money figuring out if masks work.)

The researchers combined the results of the 10 trials into a single "meta-analysis" – a review that looks at each study and figures out what they say as a whole. Their conclusion – published in Emerging Infectious Diseases, a Centers for Disease Control journal – was straightforward:

> We **did not find evidence** that surgical-type face masks are effective in reducing laboratory-confirmed influenza transmission, either when worn by infected persons (source control) or by persons in the general community to reduce their susceptibility. [Emphasis added]

(https://wwwnc.cdc.gov/eid/article/26/5/19-0994_article)

A trial published in 2015 on cloth and surgical masks used by healthcare workers in Vietnam reached an even more depressing conclusion. The study was the first randomized trial to examine the use of cloth masks, which healthcare workers in poorer countries commonly wear.

The researchers found healthcare workers who wore cloth masks were *more* likely to develop infections than those who wore surgical masks as well as a third control group who were not required to wear masks at all. The trial did not include N95 respirators, since respirators are uncommon in poorer countries and the researchers wanted to offer realistic alternatives.

But the researchers did put both masks and N95s through lab tests to see how easily particles penetrated them. They found that cloth masks stopped only *3* percent of particles, and medical masks stopped just over half. The N95s stopped 99.9 to 99.99 percent of particles.

In their discussion, the researchers wrote that the trial

> suggests HCWs [health-care workers] should not use cloth masks as protection against respiratory infection... the physical properties of a cloth mask, reuse, the frequency and effectiveness of cleaning, and increased moisture retention, may potentially increase the infection risk for HCWs.

(https://www.ncbi.nlm.nih.gov/pmc/articles/PMC4420971/)

Of course, none of these studies specifically looked at Sars-Cov-2, since they were all conducted before this year. They were also all relatively small.

If only we had a large randomized controlled trial that specifically examined whether masks protected their wearers from the coronavirus.

Now we do.

In a paper published on Nov. 18, Danish researchers reported on a trial that covered almost 5,000 people in Denmark in the spring. The trial was carefully designed and executed, with half the participants told to wear high-quality surgical masks and provided 50 for free. The other half were not asked to wear masks. Participants were followed for a month to see if they had been infected with Sars-Cov-2.

Within the month, 53 people in the maskless group had been infected, compared to 42 who wore masks. The difference was indistinguishable from chance, and suggested masks might really cause anywhere from a 46 percent decrease to a 23 percent *increase* in infections among their wearers.

The reason for the failure was not that people in the masked group didn't follow the rules, either. When they looked at only at participants who always wore masks, the researchers found an even smaller difference. Mask wearing "did not reduce, at conventional levels of statistical significance, the incidence of Sars-Cov-2 infection," the authors wrote in their discussion.

Unless future large randomized controlled trials find different results, the Danish mask study essentially should end the debate if surgical masks protect people who wear them outside hospitals.

As physicians and infectious disease professionals largely agreed until April, the answer is that they don't. Anyone who says otherwise, for whatever reason, is being untruthful – and as of Nov. 10, that group, unfortunately, includes the Centers for Disease Control.

3

But what about the second part of the promise mask advocates make: that my mask protects *you*, while yours protects *me*?

And what about the mandates that flow out of that promise – that for us to protect each other, we *all* must wear masks, even if we are not showing symptoms of Covid?

Those questions turn out to be even *more* complicated than the one of whether masks protect their wearers. For the "my mask protects you" theory to be true and universal mask mandates to make sense, several different and highly technical questions must align. Those include:

The size of the particles people exhale;

The filtration characteristics of ordinary cloth and surgical masks;

Whether people are wearing masks properly;

The number of viral particles needed to cause an infection;

The relative risk of infection inside and outside and how well the virus can survive in sunlight or harsh conditions;

The question of whether people who are infected with Covid but not showing symptoms can have sufficient viral loads to infect other people.

We don't have precise answers to all of those questions. But the answers we do have tend not to support the logic behind source control – "my mask protects you."

The theory is essentially as follows: infected people exhale the virus in both droplets and aerosols, large and small particles. A mask, even a cloth mask, can catch droplets and thus reduce the total amount of virus a person is exhaling. Plus, because large particles tend to fall to the ground quickly, masks are even *more* important when two people are close together. The reason is in that case the mask might provide some protection to the wearer, too – because it will catch droplets that the person would otherwise inhale before they hit the ground.

Intuitively, the idea makes sense. But the details are crucial.

For example, if most particles people exhale are very small, catching larger particles may not matter much. Measuring the exact size of the particles in people's breath is technically challenging. But in 2009 researchers did so. What they found is not good for mask advocates. The vast majority of particles in exhaled breath are tiny, smaller than a micron.

In the paper, called "Size distribution and sites of origin of droplets expelled from the human respiratory tract during expiratory activities," the researchers reported:

> The majority of droplets from human expiratory activities are very small, being in low micrometer and high sub-micrometer ranges. Where Papineni and Rosenthal [an earlier study] found that 80–90% of droplets were smaller than 1 μm [micron], the current study agrees, showing that these smallest particles are located within an aerosol mode, centered in the range 0.1–1 μm.

(https://www.sciencedirect.com/science/article/pii/S0021850208002036)

In basic terms, masks have almost no chance of catching most of the particles we exhale.

Of course, if larger droplets happen to hold most Sars-Cov-2 virions, then maybe masks can help even if they don't do much good against smaller particles. For many years, scientists believed large droplets *did* hold most viral particles – in part because they simply have much more room. Imagine a marble in a box – if the box is a foot on each side, it can hold the marble easily, but if it is only an inch, the marble will have to drop in perfectly.

But just as researchers can now determine the size of the particles that people exhale, they now know which particles hold virions. Again, the answer is not good for the source control theory.

In a remarkable paper published in the September 2020 issue of The Lancet: Respiratory Medicine, Dr. Kevin P. Fennelly – a pulmonologist at the National Heart, Lung, and Blood Institute – debunked the view that larger droplets are responsible for most viral transmission. Fennelly wrote:

> Current infection control policies are based on the premise that most respiratory infections are transmitted by large respiratory droplets—ie, larger than 5 μm [microns] — produced by coughing and sneezing...

Unfortunately, that premise is wrong, Fennelly explained.

Studies "that included methods to measure particle sizes have consistently found pathogens in small particles (i.e. under 5 microns)." A study of influenza patients found about two-thirds of all the virus was contained in particles under 4 microns.

Other researchers found that particles under 5 microns contained 9 times as much flu virus as larger particles. (That paper did show surgical masks cut the amount of virus found in smaller particles – a point for "my mask protects you" – but by far less than they reduced the virus in larger particles.)

"There is no evidence that some pathogens are carried only in large droplets," Fennelly wrote. Even the fact that risk rose when people were close together didn't provide much evidence for the droplet theory. Small particles also had a higher risk of infecting people at short distances.

Making matters worse, some pathogens are *more* dangerous when they spread via smaller particles, probably because smaller particles penetrate more deeply into the lungs than larger ones. Fennelly noted a breakthrough 1953 paper on anthrax that showed that single bacterial spore of about one micron was significantly more lethal than larger clumps of spores.

Fennelly did not go so far as to call masks useless – a near impossibility in the current environment – but he was lukewarm at best on their value to protect other people even in the most obvious case, when they are worn by symptomatic patients in hospitals. "Masking of patients can help to partly reduce infectious aerosol exposures to health-care workers, but are not a substitute for physical distancing and other infection control measures."

Instead, he called for a focus on improving ventilation as well as "air disinfection with ultraviolet germicidal irradiation," especially for nursing homes, where so many Covid deaths have occurred.

(https://www.thelancet.com/journals/lanres/article/PIIS2213-2600(20)30323-4/fulltext)

Further, even if masks do keep people from exhaling enough large particles to reduce the amount of virus around them substantially, and even if large and small particles are equally dangerous, and even if people wear masks properly –

Forcing everyone to wear masks will matter very little unless asymptomatic people spread the coronavirus in large numbers. Everyone agrees people who are symptomatic with a fever or cough should stay home or wear a mask if they must go out. If only sick people are wearing masks, face coverings may function as a public signal: *I don't feel well, stay away.*

But the *point* of universal mask mandates is to force people who do not feel sick to wear masks anyway, on the theory that people without symptoms can also spread the virus.

Like practically every other part of the "my mask protects you" theory, this aspect is unproven. Worse – like the advice around general lockdowns, which were never recommended before March – it has become highly politicized. Scientists including Anthony Fauci have reversed course on the likelihood of asymptomatic transmission. At a press conference in January, Fauci could not have been clearer. Asymptomatic transmission was not a threat:

> The one thing historically people need to realize is that even if there is some asymptomatic transmission, in all the history of respiratory-borne viruses of any type, asymptomatic transmission has never been the driver of outbreaks. The driver of outbreaks is always a symptomatic person. Even if there's a rare asymptomatic person that might transmit, an epidemic is not driven by asymptomatic carriers.

(https://www.youtube.com/watch?v=X1orSO094uY)

At a press conference on June 8, a senior World Health Organization scientist also said people almost never transmitted the coronavirus if they did not have at least mild symptoms. In response to a question about asymptomatic transmission, Maria Van Kerkhove, an epidemiologist and the "technical lead" for WHO's Covid-19 response team, said:

> We have a number of reports from countries who are doing very detailed contact tracing. They're following asymptomatic cases, they're following contacts and they're not finding secondary transmission onward. It's very rare.

People who were reported to be asymptomatic generally had at least mild disease, like a low fever or cough, Van Kerkhove said.

(https://www.who.int/docs/default-source/coronaviruse/transcripts/who-audio-emergencies-coronavirus-press-conference-08jun2020.pdf?sfvrsn=f6fd460a_0)

The relative lack of asymptomatic transmission shouldn't be surprising, for the coronavirus or any respiratory illness, because *symptoms and severity of illness usually rise with viral load.* As early as March, Chinese researchers reported that "our data indicate that... patients with severe Covid-19 tend to have a high viral load and a long shedding period." An August study reached a similar conclusion.

(https://www.thelancet.com/journals/laninf/article/PIIS1473-3099(20)30232-2/fulltext)

Of course, some people can show no symptoms even when testing reveals they have relatively high levels of the virus. Other studies have shown no or a small overall difference in viral loads between symptomatic and asymptomatic patients.

And computer modeling suggests that up to 40 percent of infections could come from asymptomatic cases.

But when real-world contact tracers tried to find actual evidence of asymptomatic spread of Sars-Cov-2, they are basically unable to do so. In July, the WHO noted that four studies had showed that "between 0% and 2.2% of people with asymptomatic infection infected anyone else."

(https://www.who.int/news-room/commentaries/detail/transmission-of-sars-cov-2-implications-for-infection-prevention-precautions)

The most stunning example of this came from a city-wide screening for Sars-Cov-2 in May in Wuhan, China, where the virus apparently originated. Researchers tried to test *everyone* in Wuhan. They nearly succeeded, carrying out almost 10 million tests. They found 303 people who tested positive for the virus. All 303 cases were asymptomatic. The scientists then traced 1174 close contacts of those people – and found not one had been infected. "There was no evidence of transmission from asymptomatic positive persons," they wrote.

(https://www.nature.com/articles/s41467-020-19802-w)

But the media and other public health experts immediately pushed back on Van Kerkhove's accidental honesty in the June 8 press conference. Why? Because the threat of asymptomatic transmission is critical to the argument for universal mask mandates.

If people without symptoms are very unlikely to transmit Sars-Cov-2 to others, why make them wear masks at all? The evidence is overwhelming that surgical or cloth masks don't protect their wearers, so whom exactly are the masks protecting?

Within 48 hours, Van Kerkhove and the WHO were forced to walk back their statement, at least partially. The organization tried to distinguish between "asymptomatic" and "presymptomatic" carriers – people who had just been infected and were about to get sick but hadn't yet. Those presymptomatic carriers might have a short window where they were infectious.

In reality, though Van Kerkhove's statement was in keeping with the WHO's views about asymptomatic transmission and masks. On June 5, the organization had released a statement entitled "Advice on the use of masks in the context of Covid-19." The paper ran 16 pages and included 80 footnotes and this stunning statement:

> At the present time, the widespread use of masks by healthy people in the community setting **is not yet supported by high quality or direct scientific evidence** and there are potential benefits and harms to consider. [emphasis added]

(https://www.who.int/publications/i/item/advice-on-the-use-of-masks-in-the-community-during-home-care-and-in-healthcare-settings-in-the-context-of-the-novel-coronavirus-(2019-ncov)-outbreak)

The WHO then managed to choke out the weakest possible recommendation for mask use by healthy people: "In areas of community transmission, governments should encourage the general public to wear masks in specific situations and settings."

How many caveats did WHO put on this supposed recommendation?

In a table, the paper explained that – for example – people working in countries with "limited or no capacity to implement other containment measures such as physical distancing [and] contact tracing" might "be encouraged" to wear non-medical

masks. The reason: "**potential benefit** of source control."
[emphasis added]

Just why was the WHO so lukewarm on wearing masks?

Though it runs to billions of dollars a year, the cost of forcing
healthy adults to wear disposable surgical masks will be
relatively minor for wealthy countries. And cloth masks are easy
to clean in places that have access to clean water. In poor
countries the calculus is different. Making people wear cloth
masks that cannot be easily cleaned or spend a significant part
of their income on disposable ones is much harder to justify if
masks don't work.

The WHO said as much in the report, saying governments
should consider "availability and costs of masks, access to clean
water to wash non-medical masks, and ability of mask wearers
to tolerate adverse effects of wearing a mask."

The science around masks and mask mandates has become
deeply politicized since April.

That's why two Canadian arbitration decisions about masks
from 2015 and 2018 – before face coverings became so totemic
that people who didn't wear them risked being called
sociopaths – are highly instructive.

The decisions arose from efforts by hospitals in the Canadian
province of Ontario to force nurses to be vaccinated against
influenza. The hospitals could not contractually make nurses
take the vaccine.

Instead they decreed that any nurse who refused would instead
be required to wear a surgical mask while working. Crucially, the
hospitals were mainly concerned with using masks for "source

control" – protecting *patients* from nurses who might be spreading the flu before they had symptoms.

In December 2013 the nurses' union filed a grievance against the policy. The case went to a neutral arbitrator, James Hayes. He heard thousands of pages of testimony from six expert witnesses, consulted 249 exhibits, and read more than 100 scientific papers.

In September 2015, Hayes issued a 136-page ruling saying hospitals could not make nurses wear masks. The "scientific evidence said to support the [mask mandate] on patient safety grounds is insufficient," he wrote.

Even the theory that masks could prevent droplet transmission was unproven, Hayes found:

> At best, there appears to be limited evidence of what to a layperson may seem obvious: a mask may prevent the transmission of large droplets. Two literature reviews refer specifically to "limited data" and to "the limited evidence base supporting the efficacy and effectiveness of face masks to reduce influenza virus transmission."

He went on to quote one of the experts the nurses offered:

> Coughing, sneezing and talking produce a wide range of particle sizes, all of which can be infectious. The smaller-sized particles will easily bypass the filter and facepiece of a surgical mask—and are likely to remain airborne for long periods of time.

Later in the report, Hayes noted that even the experts the hospitals had offered agreed that "there is limited evidence on the significant point of the utility of masks in reducing transmission risk."

In addition, wearing masks for long periods came with downsides, the nurses' experts told Hayes. Masks were uncomfortable, became moist, and could cause skin irritation. (One referred to a "grunge factor.")

So Hayes struck down the requirement, finding that even in hospitals – where masks are likely far *more* useful than other settings, given that they are filled with vulnerable patients and regularly have outbreaks of respiratory illness – the evidence did not support for mask mandates for healthy adults.

(https://www.canlii.org/en/on/onla/doc/2015/2015canlii62106/2015canlii62106.pdf)

The fight didn't end there. Some hospitals kept trying to make nurses wear masks. The nurses objected again. Again they won.

In a September 6, 2018 decision, arbitrator William Kaplan agreed with Hayes's ruling. In fact, Kaplan went further than Hayes, calling the evidence in favor of mask mandates "insufficient, inadequate, and completely unpersuasive." Later in his ruling, he wrote:

> The preponderance of the masking evidence is compelling – surgical and procedural masks are extremely limited in terms of source control: they do not prevent the transmission of the influenza virus.

(https://www.ona.org/wp-content/uploads/ona_kaplanarbitrationdecision_vaccinateormask_stmichaelsoha_20180906.pdf)

These arbitrators were not anti-mask. They were chosen for their neutrality. But both looked at the evidence and reached the same conclusion.

The decisions came in the context of the flu, not the coronavirus. But all the evidence we have suggests that both viruses, which are roughly the same size, are transmitted in the same way.

The theoretical evidence lines up nearly as strongly against the idea that "my mask protects you" as it does against "my mask protects me."

What about the real-world evidence?

Unfortunately, we do not currently have a study as definitive as the Danish mask trial for the source control theory. Such a trial would be very hard to run – it would require something like picking two similarly sized *cities* and requiring every healthy person in one to wear masks for a month or more while banning everyone in the other from doing so.

In the absence of such a trial, mask advocates have pointed to a more or less random series of case reports and observational data. For example, they have pointed to a CDC report showing two coronavirus-infected hairdressers in Missouri who wore masks did *not* infect 139 clients.

(https://www.cdc.gov/mmwr/volumes/69/wr/mm6928e2.htm)

The problem is that in the absence of other facts, we cannot know if the masks were the reason the hairdressers didn't infect their clients. Maybe the salon had good ventilation. Maybe the hairdressers happened not to be very infectious, since contact tracing studies show many people with Covid do not infect other people, while a small number of people appear to be so-called "super-spreaders."

Public health advocates also point to reports showing individual counties with mask mandates appeared to have slower growth in transmission rates than neighboring counties that did not. For example, a CDC report about the state of Kansas claimed that growth in positive tests was far lower in counties with mask mandates than those without.

(https://www.cdc.gov/mmwr/volumes/69/wr/mm6947e2.htm)

But this Kansas data is also much weaker than it appears at first. We don't know whether the rules translated into a major or even minor difference in mask use. More importantly, at the end of the period the CDC reviewed, the counties with mask mandates actually still had *higher* overall rates of Covid than those without.

Many, many other observational datapoints suggest that mask mandates have made no difference to the spread of Sars-Cov-2. Florida ended statewide mask mandates in late September, for example. But in the two months since, the state has had significantly slower growth in positive tests than the United States as a whole.

On a national basis, masks appear to have made even less difference. The United States is not alone in seeing huge spikes in positive Covid tests despite mask mandates and high levels of mask use. Most of Europe has had the same trend.

Epidemiologists agree that when clinical trials are impossible, real-world evidence must be nearly overwhelming to reach anything like the same level of proof. The best example comes with tobacco and lung cancer. Running a clinical trial to examine whether tobacco causes cancer would be both impossible and unethical. But heavy cigarette smokers develop lung cancer at rates 20 times those of nonsmokers – a difference that cannot be explained for any other reason. Even so, doctors and scientists argued for decades over potential other explanations before rejecting them.

In the case of the source control theory for masks, the real-world evidence is somewhere between weak and nonexistent. Yet instead of decades, public health authorities changed their collective mind on masks nearly overnight.

Meanwhile, though we don't have anything as good as the Danish study for source control, we do have the results of one real-world trial that touches on "my mask protects you." It was short, but well-run – and it too offers no joy to mask advocates.

This year, more than 3,000 Marine recruits participated in a two-week quarantine that included cloth mask wearing, social distancing, and daily temperature and symptom checks. They lived on a closed college campus which they could not leave. They did not even have access to "personal electronics and other items that might contribute to surface transmission."

Yet at the end of the quarantine, almost 2 percent of the Marines tested positive for the coronavirus – even in a group of Marines who were tested when the quarantine started to remove anyone who was already infected.

(https://www.nejm.org/doi/full/10.1056/NEJMoa2029717)

The study does not *prove* masks don't work as source control. Perhaps the Marines would have been infected at much higher rate if they had not been wearing face coverings. But an infection rate of 1 percent per week is hardly evidence masks work, especially given the many other protective measures the recruits used.

Yet despite the evidence that masks are of extremely marginal benefit at most for source control, public health authorities continue to insist on them.

The most obvious reasons are not medical but political.

The "good" reason is that masks are a visible totem that we are all working together against the coronavirus. We cannot all be physicians or nurses, but as they work to save lives, we all can sacrifice in this small way.

As Anthony Fauci said at a press conference in May, "It's not 100 percent effective. I mean, it's sort of respect for another person, and have that person respect you." He added that he wears masks "because I want to make it be a symbol for people to see that that's the kind of thing you should be doing."

(https://www.politico.com/news/2020/05/27/fauci-wears-mask-as-symbol-of-good-behavior-283847)

Of course, encouraging people to take actions that are (supposedly) symbolically valuable is different than *forcing* them. I may want to wear a pink pin to show I care about beating breast cancer, but Governor Cuomo can't make me.

At least I don't think he can, though I'm not so sure anymore.

The not-so-good reason is that making people wear masks frightens them. Frightens *us*. Masks are warnings none of us can escape. This virus is different. This virus is dangerous. This virus is *not* the flu. We had better hunker down until a vaccine is ready to save us all.

But the worst reason of all is that mask mandates appear to be an effort by governments to find out what restrictions on their civil liberties people will accept on the thinnest possible evidence. They are the not-so-thin edge of the wedge. Today, we must wear masks. Tomorrow we'll need negative Covid tests to travel between countries. Or vaccines to go to work.

I wish masks worked. I wish we didn't have to fight about them.

But they don't.

And we do.

Made in the USA
Coppell, TX
13 December 2020

44904741R00022